Do You Know Lisa? Volume 5

The series of books "Do You Know Lisa?" cover varies topics that Dr. Lisa Goins PhD, APRN, FNP-BC, RMT writes about throughout the year. Many topics are questions asked by patients and then published on the Couture Health Care website and are read globally.

Every year, Dr. Goins publishes the articles in a book during Nurse Practitioner week to promote awareness with health education and what Nurse Practitioners can do. Couture Health Care patients are given copies of the book during Nurse Practitioner week. Patients have been known to schedule their appointment the week of Nurse Practitioner week to make sure they get a copy.

Volume 5, will take a turn from the regular collection of health care articles from the year 2018 and focus on the events of why removal of a collaborating agreement/standard care agreement (SCA) is so important to the livelihood of the Nurse Practitioner. It will raise questions if this is even a legal practice, to pay for a signature so a Nurse Practitioner can work in states where this is required. Do you pay someone per contract so you can work?

What is a Nurse Practitioner?

A Nurse Practitioner can assess, diagnosis, plan, and treat patients/clients. Nurse Practitioners can prescribe medications and do minor procedures. Nurse Practitioners work in many specialties from hospital, urgent cares, clinics, and do home visits. Nurse Practitioners are nurses with advanced degrees, licenses, and board certifications.

Who is this famous Lisa?

Dr. Lisa Goins PhD, APRN, FNP-BC, RMT is the Founder and CEO of nonprofit Couture Health Care established in 2013. Mission statement: "Couturing individual patient's/client's spiritual and health care needs for best outcomes."

Starting nursing in 1989, Dr. Lisa has worked as a resident care tech, LPN, RN-ASN, RN-BSN, RN-MSN/APRN-Nurse Practitioner, RN-DNPc. She hold a Family Nurse Practitioner board certification from the ANCC.

In addition to nursing she holds non-secular Bachelors, Masters, and PhD degrees. She is license as Clergy in the State of Ohio and a certified Reiki/Teacher/Master.

In 2017, Dr. Lisa was reprimanded by the Ohio Board of Nursing for working without a physician signature on a standard care agreement (SCA) that allowed Dr. Lisa to provide care to Couture Health Care patients in Ohio.

This event has made Dr. Lisa the first Nurse Practitioner to be punished for working without a SCA in Ohio and the United States of American.

In addition to this, Ohio Board of Nursing is required by law to report to the National Practitioner Data Bank, also making her the first. Physicians' signatures are not needed to go to school, get a degree, pass certification, get a licenses, or get a job.

A signature is ONLY need to WORK in Ohio. Ohio is among several states that have laws that require this. Do note the signature to work is not free. A physician requires to be paid for their signature.

Dr. Lisa was paying the physician $500 per month ($6,000 a year) for his signature so she could work in Ohio. Do you pay someone so you can work?

Dedication:

Do You Know Lisa Volume 5 is dedicated to those who stand up, speak out, and do it anyway.

Disclaimer:

This is the fifth volume of health care and related articles that are part of the collection of *Do You Know Lisa?* The content is designed for general education for the public and as awesome as the information may be, this is never a substitute for seeing a Nurse Practitioner or health care provider.

Information:

If this book OFFENDS THEE, then put it down or give it to someone else to offend. May we suggest offending state's representatives where laws state Nurse Practitioners need a collaborating agreement and it should be removed?

Legal: Should anyone be interested in the legal documents, they are located online or at the courts that hold those records. Reference Warren County Courts, Ohio, the Ohio Board of Nursing, and the National Provider Data Bank. Everything is public but a charge will be needed for access to the information depending on the holders of the documents.

Editing:

Typos and errors do happen. My apologies in advance. Dr. Lisa views typos and errors as copy rights. So if you find one or many, thank your teachers for your education.

Thank you:

Thank you for your support, by purchasing, downloading, and reading this book. Thank you for all your support and responses to our social media sites, web page, and to our patients. Thank you for fighting to remove the SCAs in your states.

Special thank you and appreciation:

To my friends and Nurse Practitioner peers. This has not been easy and thank you for your support.

To my Children, thank you for being there and understanding when sometimes it was hard to.

To my Husband Jeffrey, thank you for everything you have done and standing with me through all the court, legal, business, heartbreaks, and when everything was so dark, depressing, and hopeless in my life, you were my light. You believe in me, that

I will always be a "nurse", and this is who I will always be.

Support:

What can you do to help? Educate yourself, your family, friends, and law makers on removing the collaborative agreement from your legal system. If you are a law maker, then implement and push forth for the removal of such laws in your state. Improve your state's health care and your public health care by providing access to full practice authority providers. Providers who can work to the full scope of their practice.

Call to Action:

I have been very public about the removal of the standard care agreement from Ohio's laws. I have been reprimanded by the Ohio Board of Nursing for working without a standard care agreement. The Ohio Board of Nursing then submitted my name to the National Practitioner Data Bank, where it will remain indefinitely.

I was the first in Ohio and US to be reprimanded for working without a paid permission slip. Make me the last Nurse Practitioner to be reprimanded under this unfair and un-American law.

Law:

Remove the standard care/collaborative agreements from all the state laws.

2018 Law is HB726 will remove the SCA in Ohio. Should this HB number change, please be vigilant and support any bill that may replace it or a similar bill in another state.

Welcome to the fifth volume of "Do You Know Lisa?" This book is the fifth book of primary health care articles written by Dr. Lisa Goins PhD, APRN, FNP-BC, RMT.

Articles have been published online per Couture Health Care's website, Twitter, LinkedIn, Google +, Facebook, and additional social media venues.

Yearly, the articles are rounded up and placed in digital and hardcopy book format, published, and made available on Amazon. Dr. Lisa hands out hardcopies to her patients every year during Nurse Practitioner week celebrated in Ohio in November every year.

Articles are written based on patients' request for information and education. Sometimes, health care events will inspire an article to be written.

Originally, this book was going to be a collection of articles but this year, the inspiration for the "Do You Know Lisa?" volume, is the need to remove the standard care agreement or collaborative agreement.

This book is divided into two main sections. The first section is explaining the background of a Nurse Practitioner's education. The second is the summarized timeline of events on how the Nursing Board became involved with the SCA.

A lot of other life stuff happened during this time of the legal issues and added in would give the reader an overwhelming understanding just how crazy life can get. Just dealing with the laws, SCA, and outcomes are plenty traumatizing enough.

"Ideas are easy, implementing them is the hard part."

~Dr. Lisa Goins PhD, APRN, FNP-BC, RMT

Nurse Practitioner Program Founder

Like any good story, it helps to understand how Nurse Practitioner evolved and why. Post World War II, the following years in the United States of America was facing a shortage of physicians. The time it took for a physician to be trained and hit the ground running, was taking too long to be implemented into the work force, and creating a huge gap in providers in healthcare.

Loretta Ford (Nurse) and Henry Silver (Physician) are the Founders of the Nurse Practitioner concept and implementation. Nurses turned into Nurse Practitioners were seen as already trained and with several years' additional training, would be able to be implemented quickly to fill needed health care roles. A program was started in 1965 and with funding moved forward in Colorado.

Eugene Stead (Physician) was also trying to get a similar program implemented. After many attempts at implementation and failure to fund, he approached the military with his idea of a Physician Assistant (PA). The PA was a two year intense version of medical school that created a mid-level entry to the physician education and met health care demands.

Both programs helped to decrease the years of becoming a provider and increased the access the health care providers to the public and military.

2018, finds both of these programs in place from the 1960s. The current key differences is that physician assistants (PA) have to work under supervision of a physician. Nurse Practitioners hold a licenses in nursing and function independently on their own. There are restrictions in some states where Nurse Practitioners are required to be supervised or have oversight of a physician similar to the PA.

In the State of Ohio, Nurse Practitioners are required to have a collaborative agreement or standard care agreement (SCA) per law.

To help the novice understand why this is important to them and to health care, first let's explain what a Nurse Practitioner and the education level needed to be a provider.

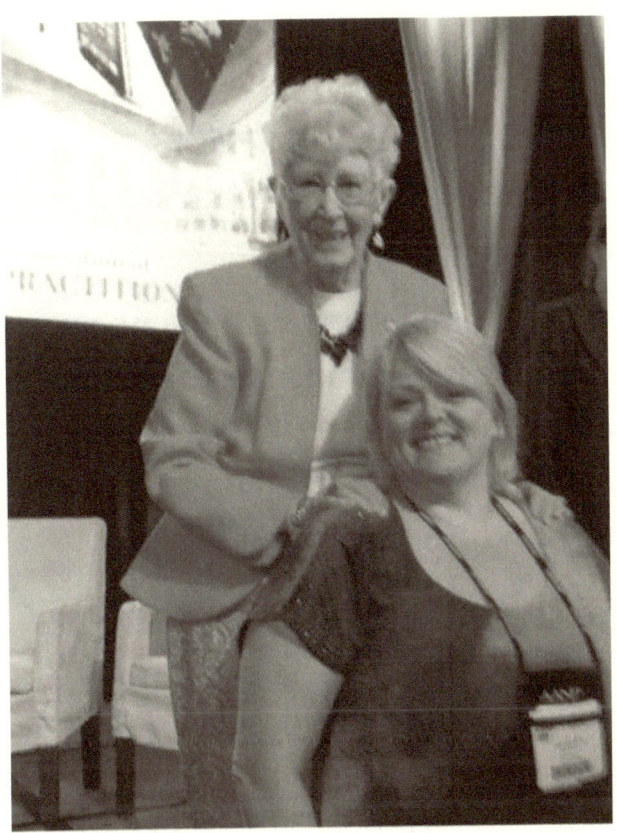

Dr. Loretta Ford and Lisa Goins

AANP Convention 2013

What is a Nurse Practitioner?

Why is the word "Nurse" used?

Let us explain the terms and how a Nurse can become a Nurse Practitioner.

Health care personnel: unlicensed staff members who care for patients in their homes, provide company and help with daily activities, and may transport to activities or appointments. This person is not a nurse.

Medical Assistant (MA): This person is trained and holds a certification or a two year degree. This person works under the supervision of any type of nurse or provider. This person can do office paperwork, give shots under supervision, and may have clinical training per classes or grandfathered since they were trained by providers. This person is not a nurse but a technician.

State Certified Nursing Assistant (STNA), Certified Nursing Assistant (CNA) or nursing assistants may have several weeks or months of training and then pass a state test to grant certification. They may work in nursing homes, in home, or hospital settings. They are staff members that do personal care and help with baths, dressing, ambulating, and eating. STNA/CNA may work under the supervision of a Licensed Practical Nurse (LPN) or Registered Nurse (RN). This person is not a nurse.

Nurses must hold a diploma/degree to be granted a licenses in the state they practice. Nurses are professionals that hold a licenses to practice.

Licensed Practical Nurse (LPN). May have one to two years of education and hold a state license to practice as a nurse. LPNs can pass medications, do vital signs, and take physician and Nurse Practitioner orders. Patient experience begins the first term or semester and many programs now require experience as an STNA before applying to school. Additional training in some states will allow LPNs to perform IV fluids and manage IV lines. LPNs are nurses and work under the supervision of a Registered Nurse (RN). This person is a nurse and will sit for an exam before granted a state license.

Example: Lisa Goins LPN (1989- retired 2006)

Registered Nurse (RN-ASN). May have a two year Associate Degree of Science in Nursing. Recognized as the Associate Registered Nurse, this nurse can administer all types of meds, blood products, and skills range from ICU to management positions. Often known as the "bedside nurse", the RNs supervise STNAs and LPNs. Patient experience begin the first term or semester. Many programs require the RN to have experience as a STNA or LPN. This person is a nurse and will sit for an exam before granted a state license.

Example: Lisa Goins ASN (earned 2006)

Registered Nurse (RN-BSN). May have a two year Associate Degree of Science in Nursing (ASN) and a continuing two years to earn a Bachelor Degree of Science in Nursing (BSN) or just earned a four year BSN. This nurse may be the charge nurse on the hospital floor, team leader of the code team, or Director of Nursing. This person is a nurse and will sit for an exam before granted a state license if they have not sat for an exam as RN-ASN.

Example: Lisa Goins ASN, BSN (earned 2008)

Masters in Nursing (RN-MSN). May have a two, three, or four year degree in the Masters in Science of Nursing (MSN) and will hold a Bachelor's degree and a Registered Nurse (RN) license in the state they practice. The requirements will depend on how the program has been credentialed. This person is a nurse with a specialty degree and already has been granted an RN license. Only a board exam is necessary for license at this level.

Example: Lisa Goins ASN, BSN, MSN (earned 2010)

Example of crediting bodies: The Accreditation Commission for Education in Nursing (ACEN) accredits all types of nursing programs. The Commission on Collegiate Nursing Education (CCNE) accredits baccalaureate and master level nursing programs.

School credentialing may have the program structured to be quarterly programs with the summers off, one class at a time, straight through the program with a holiday break until completion, meeting online for classes, or meeting at the school for instruction and training in skills. Programs may be designed to allow the BSN nurse to continue working while furthering their education.

Schools may require the student to find their own clinical sites with providers licensed in their field of study on hospital floors, urgent cares, clinics, and office settings. Tuition to schools will not cover the cost of clinical site education and students may pay additional cost to complete their education.

Nurses at the Masters level are referred as Advanced Practice Nurses (APN) or Advanced Practice Registered Nurses (APRN). Types of nurses include; Midwives (bringing babies in the world), Clinical Specialist (advanced care and treatments), and Nurse Practitioners (primary care providers).

The main difference of this level of nursing is that an APRN can diagnosis and prescribe medications and treatments. APRNs can be primary providers for patients. APRNs can work with hospitals, with provider groups, own their own companies and practices to provide health care to the public.

Example: Lisa Goins ASN, BSN, MSN, or Lisa Goins MSN

Board Certification. This exam often follows completion of the Master's prepared nurse. For the Nurse Practitioner, there are two types of Board Certification exams they may take. One is the American Association of Nurse Practitioners (AANP) or the American Nurses Credentialing

Center (ANCC). This will allow the Master's degree nurse to be called Family Nurse Practitioner (FNP). Certification from AANP will be noted as FNP-C. Certification from ANCC will be noted as FNP-BC.

Board Certifications is required in most states, including Ohio. A Nurse Practitioner will not be able to receive a license without board certification. Upon passing board certification, the Nurse Practitioner will apply to the state for an Advanced Practice Registered Nurse license (APRN). Many states require that the person at this level hold an RN and APRN licenses.

Example: Lisa Goins MSN, APRN, FNP-BC (2011)

Doctor of Nursing (DNP) or non-nursing doctoral degree (PhD). May be one to two years. This degree may include a Master's degree and allow a BSN to go to a DNP or hold a Master's degree and then return to school for a doctoral degree. This degree is often called the terminal degree or highest degree that a nurse can hold. This allows the nurse to be called a doctor. Contrary to belief and marketing, a "doctor" can be anyone who has earned a doctoral degree in any field. Many confuse a "doctor" with a physician. Depending on law, such as in Ohio, anyone using the term "doctor" must state what type of "doctor" they are to the public. An exam is offered at this level but not required for licensure or practice.

Example: Dr. Lisa Goins PhD (2013)
Example Introduction: Dr. Lisa Goins Nurse Practitioner.

A Nurse Practitioner is also known as an Advanced Practice Registered Nurse (APRN). This is the agreed term, the American Association of Nurse Practitioners (AANP) are using to unite the Nurse Practitioners across the United States of America. Currently, Nurse Practitioners have been using various versions of lettering but the AANP feels the public will be best served if the term is the same throughout the United States.

Many states are in the progress of changing. Ohio is one of them. Ohio originally called Nurse Practitioners, Certified Nurse Practitioners (CNP). To help implement the education and change throughout the state, in the years 2017-2019, Nurse Practitioners will be recognized as CNP-APRN.

Started in Nov 2019 new cycle of licensing in Ohio, the Nurse Practitioner will then be known as APRN.

Example: Lisa Goins CNP, Lisa Goins CNP-APRN, Lisa Goins APRN.

Nurse Practitioners who hold more than one state licenses may have already implemented APRN in their title.

In addition, to all the degrees and state licenses, one cannot just write prescriptions without a licenses.

The Drug Enforcement Administration (DEA) has requirements per state on what types of medications may be prescribed. Nurse Practitioners will need a licenses before they will be able to prescribe medications.

To recap, a Nurse Practitioner may have at least 6-10 years of education, 2-4 degrees or more, 3 or more licenses with various states and government agencies. Many have experience with patients their first semester of school, thus 5-9 years of experience with patients by the time they are Nurse Practitioners.

Whew. That is a lot right? Now to start working as a Nurse Practitioner.

Upon landing a job as a Nurse Practitioner, there is just one more very important piece of paper you need. Of course it depends on the state you apply and receive your licenses, and it is called a standard care agreement (SCA) or a collaborating agreement.

Oh, and depending on your state, you cannot work one day without it. Notice, I said had nothing to do with your applying to get a job, it is when you get hired, and before you can see your first patient, this paper is needed in place.

It may even need to be made into copies, sent to the board of nursing, HR, kept at your desk in case you were ever asked for it.

If you do not have this paper, you cannot work. You could even be fined, reprimanded, put in the National Practitioner Data Bank, lose your job, and have trouble finding a new job all because of this signature on this paper.

Did I mention that this paper needs to be signed by a physician? Not a Nurse Practitioner. Not any legal entity. Is this fair? Is this right? Is this legal?

When was the last time you needed a permission slip to do anything? When was the last time you were ever punished because you did not have a signature on your permission slip?

Paying to work as a Nurse Practitioner

In the United States of America, each state has different regulations on what a Nurse Practitioner can and cannot do. Currently, there are three divisions of restrictions the states have that do not involve education, licenses, or anything other than unnecessary legislation.

The first type is no restrictions to practice. These states have granted Nurse Practitioners the right to practice to the full scope of their education and licenses.

Author's note: God Bless those Nurse Practitioners in those states because they do not have the worries or the legal drama that comes with the restrictions other states have in place. The rest of this book will continue with explaining the standard care agreement (SCA) or collaborating agreement, a restriction in many states including Ohio.

The second type is a restriction by term of a collaborating agreement or standard care agreement. This is unnecessary legislation by the state that requires the Nurse Practitioner to have a contract with a physician in order to practice in their state in order to work. Each state with this law has varying stipulations that go with it.

Ohio currently has this law in place. Physicians need to hold a valid licenses in the state where the Nurse Practitioner works to sign a SCA.

States require that the Nurse Practitioner stay aware of the physician's valid licenses and keep a copy with their SCA at their job site.

Some states will require notification of the physician's name and copy of the SCA kept at the state's Board of Nursing office.

This requires the Nurse Practitioner to become an unpaid independent regulator of the physician's licenses because they need to stay compliant and keep information for the Board of Nursing.

The third type is a restriction including the collaborating agreement or standard care agreement but this time the unnecessary legislation by the state requires the Nurse Practitioner to not only have a contract but to have supervision by a physician in order to work.

Many states have or working toward removing these restrictions from their law books.

For an updated list of states, view the American Association of Nurse Practitioners (AANP) or

Google your State's Nurse Practitioner laws for more details.

Do note that the restriction to have a standard care agreement (SCA) or collaborating agreement in place to work is NOT needed for the Nurse Practitioner education or licenses. This restriction is ONLY when the Nurse Practitioner is hired to work or is self-employed.

SCAs typically require a physician to be available to a Nurse Practitioner if they have any questions to ask.

Review and audit charts for personal growth.

Sign any paperwork that the state or government requires a physician signature only, due to the restriction of state or government regulations.

Unnecessary oversight as many insurance companies will audit charts for accurate documentation to support billing and payment.

Charts reviewed by a physician does not guarantee the insurances will pay the amount billed to them.

Example: Signing a death certificate is a "physician signature only" requirement in some states. This becomes a problem when laws such as the one in

Ohio has, were ER physicians are not required to sign death certificates and the patient's primary provider needs to sign. Yet, Nurse Practitioners in Ohio cannot sign death certificates if they are the primary provider for the patient.

This agreement with a physician does not state any compensation is to be exchange for this agreement in the law but it indeed does happen. Nurse Practitioners are paying a physician to work in their own states. How does this happen?

First, a Nurse Practitioner may be hired by a company in a state with the SCA restriction. This company must provide the Nurse Practitioner with a signed SCA with a physician.

There are different formats on legal contracts that are available to the Nurse Practitioner and/or company, many provided by the state's Nurse Practitioner organizations.

Typically, to avoid legal concerns, the Nurse Practitioner contract will not state that they are paying the physician for this requirement by law.

Where the information will be found that the physician is being compensated for it, the information will be in the physician's contract.

Physicians understandably want to be compensated for their work and efforts. This includes any additional work load placed on them by the companies to sign SCAs for their co-workers.

Compensation to the physicians will often state a % of the revenue generated by the Nurse Practitioner that the company bills insurances.

This % may decrease after the Nurse Practitioner has been credentialed with the insurance companies.

The reason this happens is because the company will bill the patient under the physician's information until the Nurse Practitioner's information has been validated with the insurance company.

Example: If the company bills the insurance company $100 per patient seen and the Nurse Practitioner is seeing 3 patients per hour per day, which is 24 patients or $2,400 per day billed to the insurance company.

The Nurse Practitioner works 5 days per week and sees 24 patients each day. That week, the company would bill $12,000 to the insurance company. $12,000 x 4 weeks is $48,000 a month.

Should the physician ask for 10% of that revenue because of the SCA, which would be $4,800 per month income or $57,000 per year in additional income per Nurse Practitioner SCA?

Author's note: credentialing with the insurance companies means that the insurance company has agreed to give the Nurse Practitioner an identification number to charge the insurance company for the insurance company's customers that have been seen by the Nurse Practitioner.

Credentialing takes many months by insurance as each insurance company verifies all the education, licenses, background, and SCA if required by state to be in place and accurate.

Insurance companies also like to buck on paying the 100% to Nurse Practitioners for work completed and billed. The rates vary per insurance company and state and can be 15% to 50% less paid by the insurance company for the Nurse Practitioner's work than the same work done by the physician and billed under the physician's insurance identification.

This is an incentive for companies to try and bill under the physician's insurance numbers than the Nurse Practitioner's insurance numbers to keep revenue high. Thus, patient's charts will have both a Nurse Practitioner and Physician signature and the Nurse Practitioner signature will be omitted for billing to the insurance company to ensure the maximum revenue paid by the insurance company.

Other types of compensation to the physician for the Nurse Practitioner, instead of revenue before or after billing by the company, may be a flat % of monthly revenue generated, or an agreed upon flat rate every month per Nurse Practitioner SCA contract.

Because the lack of physicians needed to sign Nurse Practitioner SCAs, many states will allow a physician to sign from 5 to 10 SCAs. This can be very profitable to the physician. A physician could easily have up to 15 SCAs in place over several states. Each SCA bringing in several hundreds of dollars per month.

Example:

A physician decides to increase his income with SCAs. Each SCA he decides to charge $1,500 per month. This would be $18,000 per year. If he had 15 Nurse Practitioners SCAs in place, his total take for one year would be $270,000. ($18,000 x 15 SCAs = $270,000).

Second, a Nurse Practitioner starts up their own company. Before they can see and bill for their first patient, they need to have an SCA in place.

As the owner/founder of the company, there is no one to provide the physician signature needed. The Nurse Practitioner will need to begin asking physicians if they will sign an SCA. They may know of a physician or worked with a physician at a prior job who will sign their SCA.

Agreements may be agreeable to referring patients instead of monetary exchange, use of space in the Nurse Practitioner's office, to charging the Nurse Practitioner per month for the SCA.

In addition to money fee for the SCA, the physician may decide that the Nurse Practitioner needs to provide insurance coverage and other perks agreed on.

Depending on the laws in the state where the Nurse Practitioner needs the SCA, there may or not be a grace period if something happens to the physician.

People do die. Physicians do die and when they sign SCAs with Nurse Practitioners, Nurse Practitioners dies with them. This means that the Nurse Practitioner can no longer see patients. No notice to patients. No refills, no care, and no provider. Just like that, patients can have no one to care for them.

It does not matter that the Nurse Practitioner has education, valid licenses, and even a DEA licenses to prescribe medications. That SCA doesn't have a living physician signature, sorry for your luck.

Ohio's SCA

What is the standard care agreement (SCA) or collaborative agreement?

Reference: http://codes.ohio.gov/oac/4723-8-04v1

In the State of Ohio, the standard care agreement is in the law involves all Advanced Practice Registered Nurses (APRNs). In Ohio, this includes certified nurse-midwife, certified nurse practitioner, or clinical nurse specialist.

Ohio's smart APRNs understood this law and how it worked. They worked together and managed to pass a HB216 that became law in 2018. This law gave Nurse Practitioners 120 days to find someone else to replace a dead physician signature or a physician signature that needed to be replace for various reasons.

One of the biggest problems the bill had to address was the lack of physicians that were working in Ohio. There was not enough physicians to sign Nurse Practitioner SCAs. Ohio has over 12,000 APRNs that need SCAs. No SCA, no job.

Ohio has educated and licensed Nurse Practitioners that can see and take care of patients, but cannot work because of a need of a physician's signature on the Ohio state required permission slip.

Of course, just like Cinderella needed to be gone by midnight because all the magic was over, day 121 of the SCA, your freedom to practice without an SCA for 120 days is over.

Silly isn't it? A Nurse Practitioner can work 120 days or 4 months with no SCA. Wonder why they could not work the rest of the 8 months in the year?

Because if they could work one day safely, what makes 8 months so unsafe? Crazy to think that Nurses are the #1 ethical group in the United States of America but need over site from a less ranked ethical group?

Then what happens on day 121? If the Board of Nursing has been notified that your physician signature is gone, they contact you to verify if you have a SCA in place to work. If you do not, they start legal proceedings to try and take your licenses.

Author's note: If you are a Nurse Practitioner and the Nursing Board contacts you, contact your lawyer STAT. If you do not know a lawyer or have funds to pay a lawyer, contact your insurance company and file a complaint under the protection of your licenses section of the policy.

The insurance company will help you find a lawyer and they have an invested interest to find someone that will accept the rate they pay and settle the problem in a financially feasible way.

If the Board of Nursing is talking with you, they have already started a case with a file number regarding you. Just a reminder. The Board of Nursing is there to keep the pubic safe and they have lawyers who work with them to keep that true.

Currently, as of writing this book, Ohio has another bill called HB726 in place. This is to remove the SCA from the law books in Ohio.

This would allow Nurse Practitioners to work without the fear of losing their physician's signature on their SCA for any reason. This would stop the fear of what happens when day 121 comes about and they do not have a replacement signature. This prevents patients from losing their provider and companies/offices from closing.

Punishment is issued by the Board of Nursing for anyone holding a nursing license.

Board of Nursing. The Board of Nursing's job is to keep the public safe. This organization consist of a small group of people in charge. Either voted in or appointed to the job.

The Board of Nursing's job includes giving nurses their licenses or taking them away. Going to school, getting a degree, passing board exams and certifications, filling out application, background check, finger prints, and paying for the license will enable the Board of Nursing to give you a license.

To take your license away or get investigated by the Board of Nursing includes reports from the public or work place regarding harm, drugs, arrested for DUI/OUI, and so forth.

Once the Board of Nursing has decided on an action, this is followed by a fine, reprimand, suspension of license, revoking license, or other punishments based on the type of infraction of the law caused.

Author's note: In Ohio, the Board of Nursing can reprimand, fine for $500, and require 10 contact hours of education for working past 120 days without a collaborating agreement signed by a physician.

After the ruling of action, The Board of Nursing is required by law to report you to the National Practitioner Data Bank.

What is the National Practitioner Data Bank (NPDB)?

The NPDB is an organization by the US Department of Health & Human Service and currently contains 1.3 million reports.

It is required that all healthcare federal and state entities report per law. It is a Federal online repository that contains medical malpractice payments, adverse actions, health care related judgments or convictions/exclusions on health care practitioners.

Practitioners may do self-query for a fee and those that report to the data base pay a fee. NPDB is prohibited by law to change or remove any report submitted. All reports are infinite.

Reference: https://www.npdb.hrsa.gov/index.jsp for more information.

Doing the Impossible with Nothing. ~

Dr. Lisa Goins PhD, APRN, FNP-BC, RMT

Correction:

Do the IMPOSSIBLE with NOTHING.~

Dr. Lisa Goins PhD, APRN, FNP-BC, RMT

Greetings. The first part of this is book was to educate on the background of what a Nurse Practitioner is and how one goes about becoming one.

By this point you have an understanding of what a Nurse Practitioner is, SCA, Board of Nursing, and NPDB.

Now for how Dr. Lisa became the first one to be punished by the Ohio Board of Nursing with a reprimand, fine, continuing educational hours, then reported to the NPDB.

This makes her the first one ever punished for working without a standard care agreement or a permission slip. Remember, a standard care agreement has nothing to do with earning a degree, passing boards, background checks, finger prints, nursing licenses, DEA licenses…it is a permission slip to work. AND to have one for a company you start, often a PAID permission slip to work.

Author's note: The following is a time line of events. The goal of this book is to educate on why the removal of the SCA is important. Interested parties wanting to know the details may search legal documents and review them at their leisure. A lot of life happened around each of the two major events that follows in the book, but do to the overwhelming stress of just dealing with reading about the legal outcomes is enough for this book.

After working as a Nurse Practitioner for others, Dr. Lisa founded Couture Health Care to do house and office visits. It was started out with a concierge model and grew from there.

2013/October Dr. Lisa founded the company called Couture Health Care. Couture Health Care Limited was established in Ohio as a nonprofit Limited Liability Corporation (LLC). The search for a collaborating physician began.

2014/March Couture Health Care secured a soon-to-be retiring physician to collaborate that was paid no fee. The physician offered use of his office space on weekends to see patients.

2014/September Couture Health Care completed the changed from an LLC to a Corporation as part of the structure needed for the IRS nonprofit status requirement.

Ohio allowed LLCs to be nonprofits but the IRS did not grant nonprofit status to LLCs, only Corps.

Couture Health Care became a 501c3 nonprofit corporation recognized by the IRS. Dr. Lisa was considered the founder of the company, the CEO, and part of the Board of Directors for Couture Health Care.

2015/March Couture Health Care's collaborating physician contract expired. The company was unable to see any patients until a new collaborating physician could be replaced. Therefore, Dr. Lisa needed to find work outside of Couture Health Care due to no income because of the lack of a collaborating agreement per Ohio law.

2015/May 26 Dr. Lisa was hired to work at Lindenwald Medical Center. Dr. Anil Jhangiani MD rented space at Lindenwald Medical Center to see patients and here is where Dr. Lisa was introduced to him.

2015/Aug 26 Upon the 90 day mark of hiring, Dr. Lisa's employment was terminated. The excuse Lindenwald Medical Center gave, was because they could no longer afford to pay her.

2015/September Dr. Lisa meet with Dr. Jhangiani regarding a collaborating agreement regarding Couture Health Care. He agreed and was to be paid $500 per month, with the first 5 months with no payment due to there would be no income and he wished to help the company grow and become established. He was continuing to see patients at Lindenwald Medical Center but was concerned with the company staying and requested that if he need, he could see those patients at the new location.

2015/October Couture Health Care opened an office in Hamilton, OH. Funding to open the office came from donations and car title loan money. $10,000 was raised. At this time the company expanded to accepting insurance. Primary Care was to be provided with no opioids prescribed.

2016/February Couture Health Care was set to shut down the office due to no insurance company had reimbursed for any patients seen. The first payment to Dr. Jhangiani was to be made.

A "Hail Mary" attempt to save the office from closing was established, when the billing company that had failed to produce income for Couture Health Care, was done in house by staff.

After correcting the mistakes made by the billing company, clarifying information with the insurance companies, two days before the end of the

February, Couture Health Care received the first insurance claim paid and was able to remain in business. Couture Health Care continued with steady growth.

2016/September Couture Health Care established two contracts with Dr. Jhangiani upon the renewal of the prior contract.

One for the collaborating agreement with Dr. Lisa and a second one for office space for Dr. Jhangiani to see patients as Lindenwald Medical Center rental agreement was not renewed.

2017/January Couture Health Care was in talks with purchasing Lindenwald Medical Center and began interviewing Nurse Practitioners to work at the location.

2017/February Couture Health Care ended talks to purchase Lindenwald Medical Center with owner. A lawsuit was filed by the Medical Director of Lindenwald Medical Center, claiming he owned the company.

2017/April Ohio HB216 was signed into law and granted Nurse Practitioners 120 days to work with no collaborating physician in the State of Ohio.

2017/August Couture Health Care notified Dr. Jhangiani that both contracts (rental/collaborating agreement) would not be renewed.

2017/October Couture Health Care was notified that Dr. Jhangiani would be suing the company over the standard care agreement. He was not suing over the rental agreement.

The decision to post the information about the lawsuit on the website and social media was made.

This was to bring public awareness of Nurse Practitioners needing a collaborating agreement and that Nurse Practitioners who owned or founded companies paid for those agreements, so the Nurse Practitioner would be able to practice and work in Ohio and other states with similar restrictions of practice that did not have any bearing on education or licenses to work in said state.

The following is the timeline that was posted on Couture Health Care's website, Twitter, LinkedIn, Facebook, and was shared by others.

2017/October 24,
Couture Health Care was notified by Warren County Court system on October 19, 2017, Dr. Anil Jhangiani MD c/o Advanced Cardiovascular Care was suing Dr. Lisa Goins PhD, APRN, FNP-BC, RMT c/o Couture Health Care regarding lack of payment for Standard Care Agreement (SCA) of $4,000. An SCA agreement is a collaborating

agreement between a Physician and Nurse Practitioner required by Ohio law 4723 (http://codes.ohio.gov/orc/4723).

October 24, 2017 Dr. Lisa Goins PhD, APRN, FNP-BC, RMT c/o Couture Health Care is counter suing for mysterious $4,000, services rendered for onsite IT, medical visit, and delinquent rental agreement payments totaling $4,650. Couture Health Care holds bank statements of cashed checks from March 2015 to September 2017 for SCA agreement paid to Dr. Anil Jhangiani MD c/o Advanced Cardiovascular Care as stated per contracts.

Couture Health Care is a 501c3 nonprofit company recognized by the IRS and the US Postal Service, providing primary health care, education, and spiritual care/counseling located at 201 North Brookwood Ave., Hamilton, OH 45013.

2017/November A countersuit was filed to the lawsuit by Couture Health Care regarding the money owed by Jhangiani.

November 13, 2017
State of Ohio, Warren County Court, Civil and Small Clams Division

Warren County Court Case No 2017CV10000987 Magistrate's decision and order "Counterclaim is hereby ORDERED DISMISSED because it was filed by a non-attorney on behalf of a business entity which is the unauthorized practice of law". - Wm. Robert Kaufman, Magistrate Warren County Court.

For Magistrates" Decision Only:
A party shall not assign as error on appeal the Court's adoption of any factual finding or legal conclusion, whether or not specifically designated as a finding or fact or conclusion of law under Civ. R. 53(D)(3)(a)(ii), unless the arty timely and specifically objects to that factual finding or legal conclusion as required by Civ. R. 53(D)(3)(b).

The Magistrate of Small Claims Court, where it is legal to represent yourself or company without a lawyer, had decided that the company's legal and authorized person was not able to file a countersuit because they were not a lawyer.

Court date is set for Monday December 4, 2017 at 1pm at Warren County Court, Lebanon, OH.

2017/December Due to the historical event of being the first Nurse Practitioner sued in court over the standard care agreement, Dr. Lisa publicly invited everyone to attend the event. The invite was placed on the website and social media.

DECEMBER 4, 2017
You are invited to the **historical lawsuit** *of Dr. Anil Jhangiani MD c/o Advanced Cardiovascular Care vs Dr. Lisa Goins PhD, APRN, FNP-BC, RMT c/o Couture Health Care regarding lack of payment for Standard Care Agreement (SCA) of $4,000. An SCA agreement is a collaborating agreement between a Physician and Nurse Practitioner required by Ohio law 4723 (http://codes.ohio.gov/orc/4723).* **This is the first time anyone has been sued in court regarding the SCA.**

Monday December 4, 2017 at 1pm at Warren County Court-Small Claims Court, Lebanon, OH. (Directions see their website)

12/5/2017
Warren County Small Claims Court Outcome:

- *The Judge acknowledged Dr. Lisa Goins PhD, APRN, FNP-BC, RMT Goins was not a lawyer and allowed her to present for Couture Health Care due to the nature of small claims court. A dispute by the Plaintiff lawyer.*

- *The Judge added Dr. Lisa Goins PhD, APRN, FNP-BC, RMT name to the case along with Couture Health Care due to her name was mentioned and she is also the agent for Couture Health Care. Both were named in the contract but not in court filings. A correction of the Plaintiff lawyer.*

- *The Judge acknowledge that Couture Health Care was a 501c3 corporation and not an LLC. That there was no shares issued to Dr. Lisa Goins PhD, APRN, FNP-BC, RMT. A correction of the Plaintiff lawyer, stating that Dr. Goins indeed have shares of company.*

- *Exhibits A, B, C, D by the Plaintiff lawyer did not include all checks submitted to Dr. Anil Jhangiani MD. The last check for two months was omitted by the Plaintiff lawyer and was disputed.*

- *The Judge acknowledge the checks submitted in exhibit C did NOT have account information removed and ordered a court seal over information to protect information. Error on Plaintiff lawyer's submission.*

- *The Plaintiff lawyer claimed $3,500 was owed to Dr. Anil Jhangiani, not the filed $4,000.*

- *The Judge clarified the language handwritten by Dr. Anil Jhangiani with the Plaintiff lawyer because of poor copies submitted to court regarding exhibit A, page 3, section 5.*

- *The Judge granted an extension of 30 days for more evidence to be submitted.*

The Magistrate (Judge) had decided that there needed to be more evidence regarding the issues presented and asked for an extension so Couture Health Care could do this and noted that Lisa Goins, as representative of Couture Health Care, and was able to do this in Small Claims Court.

12/15/2017
Warren County Small Claims Court Filing 12/15/2017:
Couture Health Care/ Lisa Goins is requesting another hearing to review exhibit F and exhibit G information.
Exhibit F and Exhibit G submitted as evidence.

Exhibit F:
Lisa Goins ask for a permanent stay of execution of the Ohio Standard Care Agreement in court. Supporting evidence submitted:

- *United States Government's Press Release announcing Veterans Administration allowing Nurse Practitioners to work to their full scope of practice in all 50 states without a standard care agreement.*
- *4723.43 of Revised Code stating a Nurse Practitioner may work 120 days with no standard care agreement*
- *Registered Licensed (RN) in Ohio*
- *Advanced Practice Registered Licenses (APRN) in Ohio*
- *State of Ohio Board of Nursing Certication of Authority*
- *Masters Degree in Nursing*
- *Board Certification*
- *DEA*
- *NPI*
- *Butler County Police Finger Prints.*

Documents supporting Couture Health Care/ Lisa Goins

- *Articles of Incorporation*
- *Statutory agent with Ohio*
- *IRS approval letter*
- *US Postal approval letter*
- *Tax ID number*
- *PhD degree*
- *Clergy licenses*
- *Reiki/Master/ Teacher Certification*

Exhibit G:
Clarification of term "pro-rated" in Exhibit A and Exhibit G contracts.
Exhibit B clarification of checks for payment.
Clarification of services rendered to Anil Jhangiani by Couture Health Care that have not been paid.

Pending Hearing Date at this time. (Post on Facebook, people reached 9756, engagements 2,557)

2017/December Dr. Lisa meets with a physician near Columbus, Ohio to discuss collaborating agreement. Ask for a percentage of the company for his service. Couture Health Care Board Members meet. The company does not offer stock to members, thus a percentage of the company would not be paid. The physician responds by removing the offer.

2017/December Dr. Lisa has been in talks with a physician for several months regarding a collaborating agreement. Agrees at this time but has now decided he wants $1,500 per month and payment needs to begin at the date of signing. He refers Dr. Lisa to contact his Lawyer for the contract. Couture Health Care Board Members meet and decide the amount is not financially feasible and does not move forward with the offer.

It was no escaping the public's eye that there was an issue with the SCA and Couture Health Care. After many thousands of views on social media regarding the legal issues, the Ohio Board of Nursing was alerted there may be a problem with a Nurse Practitioner working without an SCA. The determination of the new law of 120 days was no implemented but the Ohio Board of Nursing did not know if it had been violated or not.

12/21/2017
Ohio Board of Nursing Requesting SCA
Ohio Board of Nursing has request a copy of the Standard Care Agreement, exhibit A and exhibit B from Couture Health Care on Lisa Goins. Documents of exhibit A, B, and email correspondence of updating the Ohio Board of Nursing of SCA physician name faxed to their office per 4723 of the Ohio Revised code.

Per Ohio Board of Nursing Disciplinary Complaint Protocol, compliance protocol number: C-PRO-001, Board updated on May 17, 2017. Page 4 of 20 pages, (n.) Complaints based on failure to maintain a standard care arrangement: Reprimand, Fine, and continuing education Consent Agreement if there are no additional violations. (6,273 people reached on Facebook)

Nothing involving the law and courts ever resolves quickly. Couture Health Care had expected a resolution of the lawsuit involving the money for the SCA, but the hearing of additional evidence was not scheduled until February. It was not clear if the SCA was still binding, in place, concluded, or completed to Couture Health Care, as it was questionable the moneys requested may be extend longer than the contract had stated.

02/26/2018
Hearing of additional evidence of exhibit F and exhibit G and ruled:
 "Take it under advisement and will issue a written order." -Judge Kaufman, Warren County, Ohio. Plaintiff lawyer was present, plaintiff did not show in court.

Couture Health Care continued with their expansion plans. Since the purchase of Lindenwald Medical Center did not work out, the decision to move across the border to Kentucky was decided. Kentucky does not require an SCA with a physician for working in Kentucky and not prescribing opioids.

2018/March 2 Couture Health Care expands to a second location in Florence, Kentucky.

2018/March 5 Ohio Board of Nursing request more information and that there has been a case opened. (Case #17-006729).

At this time, it had not been clear that the Ohio Board of Nursing had opened up a case and was implementing it.

After several causal request via email for material, Dr. Lisa requested that the emails be on official letterhead, as it was viewed, this may not be the real Ohio Board of Nursing emailing. It could indeed, be a prank or phishing email.

An email on letterhead was returned to Dr. Lisa with a case number on it. It was the real Ohio Board of Nursing and they were interested in pursuing legal action regarding lack of an SCA.

The Ohio Board of Nursing never sent any letters in the mail. They only communicated via telephone and emails.

Dr. Lisa reached out to her insurance company and activated her licenses protection coverage. The insurance company reached out to the insurance company ranked in the top lawyers by US News, to the company in Columbus, OH. The lawyer's office is walking distance to the Ohio Board of Nursing.

Not everything posted on social media is received well by everyone and not everyone agrees. Responsibility for what is said and acceptance of such information, can bring a lot of pain, enemies, and backlash not foreseen.

Dr. Lisa was asked to curtail the social media broadcasting to help the law team get the upper hand on dealing with the first ever case in Ohio with a Nurse Practitioner and SCA. To get the word out and not piss off the law team, Dr. Lisa posted the following on Facebook.

2018/March 8 *My lawyer team told me that if anyone asked about the Ohio Board of Nursing investigation of me due to the lawsuit about the standard care agreement that I lost, to refer their questions to them. Meanwhile, fight for Full Practice Authority in all 50.*

Meanwhile, Jeff Goins felt something more should be done and with Dr. Lisa's permission, wrote up a Change.org petition and circulated it. Many felt that Dr. Lisa should had penned it but did not because of the request from the lawyers.

2018/9 March Change.org petition for "End of Standard Care Agreement (Collaborating Agreement) for Nurse Practitioners. (10/29/2018- 1,696 signatures)

Dr. Lisa felt more should be done at the government level and felt the only possible way to get rid of the SCA in all requiring states, was to ask the President. It may be possible with a stroke of a pen, that all the SCAs would be deemed non-American.

2018/March 12 Dr. Lisa emailed the President of the United States of America regarding to end the SCA for all states.

After much waiting, the Magistrate's decision arrived in March. There was no cheering at Couture Health Care. The Magistrate had decided to award the physician the maximum amount in the SCA case. Technically, making it legal to pay for a SCA signature needed to work in the state of Ohio.

3/12/2018 MAGISTRATE'S DECISION- JUDGMENT AWARDED IN FAVOR OF PLAINTIFF AND AGAINST DEFENDANTS, COUTURE HEALTH CARE AND LISA GOINS, IN THE AMOUNT OF $3500 PLUS COSTS AND INTEREST FROM THE DATE OF JUDGMENT.

Couture Health Care Board Members meet and with no SCA signature possible, paying for one was too expensive, and hiring another Nurse Practitioner was neither possible, the following was decided.

2018/March 20 Couture Health Care Board members meet and vote to close Hamilton, Ohio office by end of April and relocate to Kentucky. No SCA is needed in Kentucky for Nurse Practitioners who do not prescribe opioids. Couture Health Care Patients will be contacted, offered last visit for prescriptions, and given access to charts.

Closing Office: Unlike a Nurse Practitioner who loses their job because of not having a signed collaborating agreement, Nurse Practitioners with offices need more time than just cleaning out their desk and leaving.

The unemployed Nurse Practitioner would then need to start job hunting. Jobs are not plentiful and it takes months to find one, interview, and many months before insurance credential the Nurse Practitioner in the new job.

Owning/Founding a company. Add this to what it takes to start up and grown the company. Then, shut it down.

As with any startup of an office takes weeks, so does closing an office. A health care office takes a bit more time than a regular business office due to all the contracts and restrictions in place. Notices have to be given, contracts terminated with possible legal outcomes, and patients need to be contacted.

Terminating patient relationships with a provider varies in states but patients need to be notified, given prescriptions if applicable, and access to records/charts. Referrals may not be possible if there is no other provider who takes patient's insurance. This was the case with a large percentage of Couture Health Care's patients. No one else was taking their insurance.

Contracts that are terminated are rental/option to buy building, telecommunications, each billing company insurance contracts, vaccine programs contracts, and so forth. Equipment needs to be schedule for pick up or returned to said company and it may be on their schedule, not your schedule.

State vaccine programs require the vaccines to be relocated when an office closes. The problem with Couture Health Care's vaccines was that the State of Ohio was having trouble finding someone to accept the vaccines because many local offices had already terminated their contracts and relocated their vaccines because they were not taking insurance that covered payment. Vaccines are not cheap. One vaccine can be $20-$150 per. A box can easily be several hundreds of dollars. It is not uncommon for providers to have five to ten thousand dollars in vaccines on hand to give out to patients.

Storage/downsizing/relocating or closing an office requires getting rid of equipment by selling, donating, or and so forth. Moving in may have been exciting but moving out is as relaxing. There is now a deadline to be off the premises.

Security needs increase. As the office is shutting down, risk for robbery, breaking in, people thinking they now have access to the office who do not, will be cause for concern.

Thus, unlike cleaning out your desk when as an employee, running the company is a lot different with a shutdown process.

Just when it cannot any worse. The Ohio Board of Nursing actually sent a letter, via the local Sheriff, and it was a subpoena for Dr. Lisa.

2018/April 9 Subpoena by Ohio Board of Nursing.

Couture Health Care began shut down and closure of the Hamilton office.

Ever been to a funeral visitation? How about one that last weeks? Patients were devastated. They had lost their provider over a signature.

2018/April 25 Couture Health Care will be moving office equipment out of the building today and donating it to Resource (Habitat for Humanity).

2018/April 28 Couture Health Care closes Hamilton, OH office.

2018/May 4 Couture Health Care's Florence, Kentucky office open house was held.

Meanwhile the electric bill has to be paid. The electric company does not take IOUs. They shut you off. Dr. Lisa sent out her CV online "internet land" and a company contacted her. Hiring her part-time.

2018/May 29 Dr. Lisa accepts a part-time job with IMA/QTC to conduct USA Veteran disability evaluations. QTC won the USA Government contract and was expanding into the Cincinnati, OH area.

2018/July American Association of Nurse Practitioners conference state there are now 248,000 Nurse Practitioners in the United States of America.

It takes time to grow an office from nothing. Doing nothing with the impossible, becomes the impossible.

2018/July 23 Couture Health Care closes Florence, Kentucky office due to low revenue.

After much back and forth with the Ohio Board and Nursing, the Consent Agreement was formatted. Just like all legal paperwork, you will not get everything you wanted, and sometimes it is the better of two evils.

The Ohio Board of Nursing demanded the paperwork be sent on July 28 to be in time for the July meeting. Even though it was sent timely, the Ohio Board of Nursing did not stamp it received, thus it was not part of this meeting.

The Ohio Board of Nursing only meets every two months to conduct business. The paperwork would sit for two months.

2018/July 28 Consent Agreement with Ohio Board of Nursing signed by Dr. Lisa and Lawyer. (Signed by Ohio Board of Nursing 9/27/2018)

Dr. Lisa has been in talks with IMA regarding increasing hours from part-time to full time. A contract is sent to Dr. Lisa.

2018/September 26 IMA emails contract to increase hours with IMA from part-time to full time. Signed and emailed back.

Ohio Board of Nursing meeting end of September, confirms the consent agreement placing all the terms into action. Dr. Lisa nor her lawyer was privy to the meeting and were not notified of the outcomes.

2018/September 27 Ohio Board of Nursing meeting.

Dr. Lisa updates her employer of the reprimand and need of completing ten contact hours for the Ohio Board of Nursing. Currently, Dr. Lisa has two SCAs. One with IMA and one with QTC, both for the same work.

2018/October 5 Dr. Lisa emails IMA/QTC regarding Ohio Board of Nursing reprimand and fine.

2018/October 9 IMA puts Dr. Lisa on leave for a week until QTC board meeting can decided on work status regarding the email sent about the reprimand from the Ohio Board of Nursing.

2018/October 3 postmarked (received Oct 12) Ohio Board of Nursing sends letter stating "This concerns the post-disciplinary monitoring of your September 27, 2018 Consent Agreement with the Ohio Board of Nursing (Board). The Board will be monitoring your compliance in meeting the terms and restrictions of the Consent Agreement. Confirmation of $500 fine to be paid in three months, in addition to requirements of licensure renewal and national certification, 4 hours professional accountability and legal liability, 4 hours disciplinary actions, and two hours Ohio Nursing Law and Rules.

2018/October 2 postmarked (received Oct 12) NPDB sent papers states on 10/1/2018; Initial Action: Publicly available fine/monetary penalty and reprimand for censure. Basis for Initial Action: Practicing beyond the scope of practice. Violating of federal or state statutes, regulations or rules.

2018/October 12 Dr. Lisa completes the contact hours per consent agreement.

2018/October 15 IMA notifies Dr. Lisa that she will be on leave until March when credentialing can be re-verified.

2018/October 15 Certified Mail to Ohio Board of Nursing a check for $500 and copies of required classes certificates completed. Lawyer sent copies of check and class certificates.

2018/October 17 IMA emails Dr. Lisa letter of separation of employment.

2018/October 19 Dr. Lisa at the Ohio Association of Advanced Practice Nurses Conference, Columbus, Ohio. Supporting Ohio HB726 removal of the SCA

2018/October 23 QTC special recognition for executional customer service scores and positive Veteran feedback on Customer Service Surveys for the Third Quarter. "Lisa Goins, Nurse Practitioner, Ohio"

2018/October 31 Lawyer notifies Dr. Lisa that Ohio Board of Nursing has received check and contact hours per consent agreement.

The information will be brought up at the next Ohio Board of Nursing meeting at the end of November. Post meeting, the information will be updated in the Ohio Board of Nursing and NPDB.

2018/November Happy Nurse Practitioner Week!

What happens now?

Good questions. Very traumatizing events to live through. Like many Nurse Practitioners, I want to go to work and take care of patients. Sure it would be cool to be famous and know that future nursing students will have to read about Flo, Clare, and Lisa, but those were just supposed to be daydreams not reality. Famous indefinitely per NPDB.

The reality is now to fight to remove standard care agreements from all the states. As you can already see, I was the first one and I want to be the last one punished for going "rouge". If I can work 120 days, I can certainly work 365 days…well 364, I try not to work on my birthday.

We vow to do no harm but the standard care agreement does harm.

SCAs harms the Nurse Practitioner by limiting their scope of practice.

SCAs cost financially with fees and perks, such as having to pay malpractice coverage for that permission slip.

Malpractice insurance is several thousands of dollars on top of paying for a signature.

SCAs harms businesses that have to pay for the signature.

SCAs kills small businesses.

SCAs can shut down business or prevent them from opening up.

SCA kills health care access to qualified professionals. Especially, killing business and health care with Nurse Practitioners willing to work and care for the public in areas where others aren't willing to be or serve.

My goal when the office was opened in Hamilton was to be there 20 years. I have already lived in this area for 25 years. My kids have gone to the public school system here and the local university. My oldest serves in the US Navy and my favorite Son-in-Law serves in the US Navy.

I understand my community and their needs. I know why the 911 dispatch was removed from our city because of lack of funds. I created Couture Health Care memory cards and educated my patients on calling 911, what to say, why to say it, and to expect a response in 15 minutes.

I educated my patients on to watch when the hydrants were flushed to avoid getting sick. How to know how to look for water pressure drops in their home because we no longer have a city paper or a city TV that has everyone watches because funding was loss.

I educated on the opioid crisis by not prescribing opioids and patients came to Couture Health Care because of this. Patients didn't want to be "jumped" for their prescriptions by drug seekers. Many had family members who passed from drug overdoses.

I educated on the NARCAN programs that gave our city money and watched the fire department pass my office windows, answering calls for overdoes. Then our local sheriff saying tax payers just cannot afford to keep it up the free service that had run out of money and turned toward tax payers to pay. After all, hard to argue when trucks need gas and people have to pay the electric company.

Patients came in for referrals for community mental health and waiting times increased because of services shutting down for lack of funding. Could we do anything to help? We did by finding working with the local community in streamlining the process for patients. Educated on the programs.

We accepted Medicaid patients, when a lot of the surround providers, had sold out to the major networks buying up all the provider offices around us. Couture Health Care became an island, independent of everyone else.

We worked with patients who lived in the real world. Call us and tell us you are among the living, let us know you are stuck in traffic, reschedule your appointment so someone else can have your slot. Flat tires, traffic jams, picking sick kids up, and real things happen to real people. Couture Health Care understood, it has happened to us too. We tried to work with people, after all we had planned to be open 20 years. We had time. Or so we thought.

The standard care agreement has too much power over a company and Nurse Practitioner. It is has no real bearing on the care patients receive. It does bring financial gain to the physician.

Truly, the Ohio Board of Nursing reprimand? $500 fine? Not nearly the harsh punishment as having to call and tell your patients good-bye. Ever been to a funeral visitation? How about one that was weeks long? Everyone I saw, I had to say good-bye. Some were angry, sad, and sorry for me. Some cried on my shoulder and others "fell out" in the waiting room or exam room upon hearing. How could I quit them? It was not fair. I agreed. It was not fair. And after I saw the last patient, I decided I could no longer wear black for the longest of time. The five stages of grieving had to end eventually, or so I hoped.

No, paying $500 and doing some contact hours that had nothing to do with working without a standard care agreement was easy punishment. Saying good-bye to my patients was the real punishment.

See, I still live here in this city. I pass my old office that is still up for sale. I see my patients on their jobs where I am a customer. I did not go into hiding online. I remained vocal. I am still fighting. I refuse to shut up and sit down.

I still remain vocal. I still attend the Nurse Practitioner meetings, write on the online forums, and I still support removing the standard care agreement. After reading this book, hopefully you will too.

Thank you for your support.

Now you know Lisa and that she continues to fight for the removal of the standard care agreements in the United States of America.

Remember, Dr. Lisa was the first one to be punished by the board of nursing for working without a standard care agreement. Help make her to be the last one.

If not, there will be more Nurse Practitioners to suffer lack of a permission slip for various reasons and patients will lose their primary provider.

End the SCAs that hurts our American Health Care.

Afterthought

So let us hypotheses about the future of Nurse Practitioners. Where will we be in the next several years? The future holds planned missions to the Moon and Mars in the years 2020 and so forth.

We have privation of space companies offering trips in the next several years. Besides the people needed to get us there and bring us back, ever space ship has a sick bay. We will need to be on it.

It is currently, 2018 and we will be celebrating Nurse Practitioner week across the USA. The future is looking exciting. We are nearing on 300,000 Nurse Practitioners. Add in the APRNs of all types, and certainly we are at these numbers now. There are over 115,000 Physician Assistants in 2018 and over 1,000,000 Physicians.

We all agree that Physicians are needed but we have two programs with 5 decades of proof that we can trim the fat from lengthy Physician education and get people hitting the ground running faster. Offering multiple ways to get to the finish line has always improved the odds that there will be more successful providers for health care.

Of course there are variants in each program but the core education is the same and applying pressure to stop blood, give pain medication, and comforter are similar in each field of study.

Now we need streamline the core education and we need to add skills that can be used on world, off world, and on orbiting stations, ships, and on the equipment to get us there and back. We will need all the knowledge we have now and the future education, to meet those lower gravity sick bays and new medical establishments off the planet Earth.

Programs need to be core education with training. Memorization is great for the test but we need muscle memory to kick in when codes happen to override panic. Do we really need hours and hours of residency and clinical to say someone is ready to hit the ground running? Remember, no one is coming to rescue you off world. You are it.

Everyone will have basic knowledge of basic life support and recuse but the new medical personnel may be scrubbing in to assist the robot in surgery. The robot may be programmed or operated by remote. There will be new skills, medications, and treatments that may be local to a planet, moon, or no gravity. Current skills that we are just now creating and envisioning the need to know. Many skills that will be adapted later out of necessity or knowledge learned.

We need people that can meet these needs. Someone who can be trained efficiently, quickly, and implemented into the working environment.

Not just someone who can pass the test from memory but someone who can pull their own weight because they are crossed trained in all the skills we have now and future skills. Not a specialty person. A multi-specialist person.

There is certainly no need for supervision, oversight, or standard care agreements in the future. We need these new providers (whatever name we decide on later to call this person), will need all the skills of surgeon, bedside of a nurse, ability to work as a team but the autonomy to make those decisions with the independent and support to stand by those decisions.

This is our future and if I get there first…be it the Moon, Mars, space station in orbit, there will be full practice autonomy because I believe health care is necessary. I believe we can do it.

In conclusion, we will merge the practitioner skills and education, implement new education and training for off world, and develop a new provider who is cross trained and multi-skilled to meet this new need.

I feel we can do this in less than four years, not an easy four years but well trained, educated years to meet the need.

Meanwhile, we will take our current providers and give them the training to meet the needs of the future sick bay.

And our future is now.

www.ingramcontent.com/pod-product-compliance
Lightning Source LLC
Chambersburg PA
CBHW031541210526
45464CB00003B/1097